Fast Revision for the MRCPsych CASC Exam

Don't Panic!

GIDEON FELTON
Specialty Registrar, General Adult Psychiatry
St Mary's Rotational Training Scheme

Radcliffe Publishing
London • New York

Radcliffe Publishing Ltd
33–41 Dallington Street
London
EC1V 0BB
United Kingdom

www.radcliffe-oxford.com
Electronic catalogue and worldwide online ordering facility.

British Library Cataloguing in Publication Data
A catalogue record for this book is available from the British Library.

ISBN-13: 978 184619 528 0

The paper used for the text pages of this book is FSC certified. FSC® (The Forest Stewardship Council®) is an international network to promote responsible management of the world's forests.

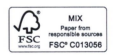

Typeset by Pindar NZ, Auckland, New Zealand
Printed and bound by TJI Digital, Padstow, Cornwall, UK

Contents

Preface

One of the best ways to prepare for any practical examination is to anticipate the range of likely scenarios that you will encounter. There is a limited range of scenarios within each subspecialty of psychiatry that can be examined. For example, within the field of substance misuse, you can anticipate the following scenarios:

1 eliciting signs and symptoms of alcohol/opiate addiction

2 short- and long-term management of opiate/alcohol/benzodiazepine addiction

3 management of relapse into addiction.

When you have developed model answers for each scenario, you are then more likely to enter the examination arena confidently. You will feel clinically 'armed and ready', which will allow you to focus more on your communication skills.

The purpose of this book is to anticipate a set of likely scenarios within each subspecialty. There will be both single-item scenarios and linked ones. Linked scenarios, denoted by **a** and **b** prefixes involve testing two different aspects within the same scenario. For example, part **a** may ask you to interview the patient with the purpose of eliciting signs of a psychiatric disorder, and part **b** may be a discussion of the management of the psychiatric disorder elicited in part **a**. You should treat the linked scenarios as two separate stand-alone scenarios because different aspects are being tested.

As there is sufficient time, actual CASC questions will try to examine several scenarios simultaneously. When faced with this, you need to unravel how many scenarios are being examined in a particular question and which are the most important. The 'instructions to candidates' rubric will guide you. For example, you may have to interview an acutely unwell patient with schizophrenia who has command hallucinations. In this case the two scenarios are (1) eliciting psychopathology and (2) assessing risk – both areas need to be covered equally well in your response.

In the examination you will receive a limited range of instructions. You can accurately predict that instructions will be either:

1 interviewing a patient to elicit signs and symptoms of a psychiatric disorder

2 discussion of the management of a psychiatric disorder with:

   a the patient

   b a relative

   c another professional.

3 discussion of new management when the original management plan fails

4 explaining management options that may make you unpopular with the listener, e.g. being detained under the Mental Health Act, or electroconvulsive therapy (ECT)

5 explanation of complicated management options, e.g. psychotherapies.

This book contains a set of possible scenarios within each subspecialty, together with a set of instructions that are likely to appear with each scenario. It is impossible to make this list totally comprehensive. Instead, this book should be used to structure your revision and give you a sense of control over the examinable syllabus.

Each scenario is followed by a set of 'musts' – things that a candidate has to do to perform well in this scenario. Each answer contains a discussion, where teaching points are outlined.

Gideon Felton
January 2011

About the author

Gideon Felton is Specialty Registrar in General Adult Psychiatry on the St Mary's Rotational Training Scheme. His special interests include prison psychiatry and substance misuse. He enjoys a strong academic and professional working relationship with Northamptonshire Healthcare where he has previously worked as a Staff Grade. Prior to studying medicine, he studied mathematics. When not engaged in psychiatry and family life, he captains the social rugby team at Old Millhillians RFC.

List of contributors

Dr Ian Treasaden
Consultant Forensic Psychiatrist
West London Mental Health NHS Trust

Dr Shamir Patel
Specialty Registrar
West London Mental Health NHS Trust

Dr Alexis Bowers
Consultant Psychiatrist
Acute Adult Services
Hertfordshire Partnership NHS Foundation Trust

Dr Olivier Van de Broucke
Consultant Psychiatrist
Child and Adolescent Mental Health Services
Hertfordshire Partnership NHS Foundation Trust

Acknowledgements

I would like to thank my wife Selma, my children Hannah and Harris, my parents, siblings, Pete R, Max CK, Nigel S and Phil S whose support has been immense.

1 Substance misuse

1a   David Hill, a 39-year-old, attends your substance misuse clinic. He is concerned about his alcohol consumption as he has lost his job and has broken up with his partner. He wants to stop drinking and is sober now. He has never been in treatment.

INSTRUCTIONS TO CANDIDATES
Assess Mr Hill for alcohol dependence.

This is about assessing the difference between alcohol dependence and alcohol-related problems.

Musts

1 Assess for:

   a the time he starts drinking

   b whether he has a narrow drinking repertoire (same drink/ same time/same place)

   c the presence of withdrawal symptoms

   d whether he experiences relief of withdrawal symptoms when he drinks

   e any drink-seeking behaviour – drinking being the most important activity of his day

   f any return to previous drinking pattern after a period of abstinence

   g the amount he drinks and whether he needs more alcohol to achieve same effect

   h whether he uses illicit drugs

   i whether he has any medical problems associated with drinking, e.g. ulcers, pancreatitis.

2 Try also to assess his previous drinking history, and any previous detoxifications and reasons for relapse.

3 Inquire about his motivation to change, i.e. what makes him want to stop drinking and what makes him not want to stop? What barriers to stopping does he see?

Discussion

The context of this scenario is a patient seeking elective help for his alcohol problem in a non-acute setting. Therefore the most important thing is to establish the degree of his physical dependence and his motivation to stop drinking. Use of CAGE would be inadequate. You are not assessing cognitive function in this assessment although this can be examined.

Notes

1b You establish that Mr Hill is physically dependent on alcohol. Discuss treatment options with him.

Musts

1 State that he must not stop drinking suddenly as he risks alcohol withdrawal.

2 Mention there is a role for an elective inpatient detoxification programme with coordinated aftercare.

3 Explain that entering a detoxification without adequate aftercare follow-up will increase risk of relapse.

4 Mention the role of regular meetings with key worker prior to inpatient detoxification.

5 Mention what happens during his inpatient stay – the roles of chlordiazepoxide and vitamins.

6 Mention the role of acamprosate and disulfiram.

7 Mention the role of rehabilitation post detoxification, i.e. residential or non-residential rehabilitation, and the place for structured day programmes to occupy patients constructively after detoxification to minimise relapse.

8 Mention role of other ancillary organisations, e.g. Alcoholics Anonymous.

Discussion

This scenario is testing the candidate's knowledge of how alcohol addiction is managed. If the patient is in delirium tremens, then this warrants emergency admission under the medical team for a medical detoxification. The disadvantage of a medical detoxification is that there is insufficient time to arrange adequate aftercare.

Therefore, in a non-urgent case, the patient would be given a specific elective date in the future to have his detoxification so that aftercare can be arranged. Aftercare is very important and the patient should try to enrol in a rehabilitation programme when the detoxification programme is finished. The patient is at the highest risk of relapse when he has just finished his detoxification.

Non-residential rehabilitation usually includes attending a structured day programme with occupational therapy. This is beneficial for patients who have good social supports at home. There is a role to play for groups such as Alcoholics Anonymous and Al-Anon as well.

Notes

2a You work for an outpatient drug misuse service. You see Mark Griffin, a 25-year-old intravenous (IV) heroin user, who attends outpatients as he wants to break his habit. He uses heroin to the value of £50 per day and has done for 6 months. He has no prior knowledge of treatments. He is in full-time employment and he has been open about his drug problem to his employers who are supportive about his treatment.

INSTRUCTIONS TO CANDIDATES

Discuss short- and long-term treatment options with Mr Griffin.

This is about knowledge of addiction treatments.

Musts

1 Explain that there are two different medications that can be used for substitute prescribing, with the aim of reducing withdrawal symptoms.

2 Explain that methadone is easier to use to begin with, given the amount he is using, so that the short-term objective would be to get him started on methadone. (Subutex is better if usage is less than half a gram per day.)

3 Explain the risks of using heroin on top of methadone.

4 Explain the risk of using alcohol and benzodiazepines with methadone – potential fatal overdose.

5 Explain the need for titration of methadone. This will take place over several days. He must try to attend the clinic in a state of 'withdrawal' and then he will be given a dose of methadone. The aim is to establish what dose of methadone will be sufficient to prevent withdrawal symptoms.

6 Explain that once an adequate dose of methadone is achieved, the next step is to try several gradual reductions.

7 Explain that prognosis is helped by regularly meeting with his key worker.

8 Explain that good general health measures, e.g. exercise, are important.

9 Explain that there are support groups for those with opiate problems that hold meetings in the evenings.

Discussion

This patient has had a relatively short habit and is new to treatment. It is important to explain the role of substitute prescribing and that it can take several days to establish the correct dose of methadone that he would need to prevent the 'cold turkey' symptoms of opiate withdrawal.

The patient will need to come to the clinic on a Monday in a state of withdrawal and he will be given a dose of methadone in the morning and a dose of methadone in the afternoon. His withdrawal state would be measured objectively. Then the patient will have his daily methadone dose calculated based on how much methadone is needed to stop his withdrawal symptoms.

In this case, methadone would be more appropriate than Subutex as he is using more than half a gram per day. It is also important to emphasise the role of non-pharmacological treatments such as groups and regular meetings with key workers.

Notes

2b Mr Griffin started on 80 mg methadone daily on supervised consumption (the pharmacist sees him taking the methadone), but after four weeks his attendance at the clinic has become less frequent. Finally, after having missed three consecutive appointments, he arrives at the clinic distressed and states that he wants to re-engage with treatment.

INSTRUCTIONS TO CANDIDATES

Try to establish the cause of the patient's distress and discuss management options with him. Do not ask whether he has been involved in any criminal activity. Do not assess his mental state.

This is about establishing the causes of relapse and initiating appropriate plans.

Musts

1 Ask about any adverse circumstances or social stressors.

2 Ask about barriers to picking up his methadone scripts.

3 Ask about whether he has picked up his methadone scripts regularly.

4 Ask if he has had a problem with pharmacists dispensing the methadone.

5 Ask if this methadone dose has been sufficient in stopping withdrawal symptoms.

6 Ask if he has been using heroin on top of the methadone.

7 Ask about concomitant alcohol or benzodiazepine use.

8 Your management will depend on your findings. Either:

a he has been using heroin on top of the methadone and has relapsed (in this case, he will have to start again with a re-titration)

b he has been using alcohol and the pharmacist has refused to dispense (in this case, he will have to have an alcohol detoxification prior to re-titration)

c he has missed his scripts and has been maintained purely on illicitly obtained opiates (in this case, he will have to start again with a re-titration).

Discussion

Relapse into illicit opiate use is not uncommon and often associated with social stressors and problems with picking up methadone scripts. Frequently these patients get lured back into illicit drug use through social pressures and this results in disengagement from treatment. These patients then have to rely on illicit opiate misuse to prevent the 'cold turkey' symptoms of withdrawals. These patients need to have their methadone dose recalculated based on their current pattern of opiate use.

Another reason for relapse is concomitant alcohol misuse. Pharmacists will not dispense methadone to patients if they appear intoxicated and therefore such patients often find it difficult to obtain legal methadone, resulting in a need for illicit heroin. In this case, the patient should have an alcohol detoxification prior to starting methadone again.

Notes

2 Schizophrenia

3 You are seeing 25-year-old Lee Oakes in your emergency clinic. He attended his general practitioner (GP) this morning who referred him to you. He has had one admission to hospital four years ago following a psychotic episode. He had no contact with psychiatric services in the last two years. He is in distress because he believes he is a 'paedophile'. He states that everyone knows he is a paedophile and that everyone is talking about him being a paedophile.

INSTRUCTIONS TO CANDIDATES
Carry out a mental state examination of Mr Oakes. Do not discuss management.

Musts

1 Ask him how and when did he discover he was a paedophile.

2 Ask if he has done anything to warrant being called a paedophile.

3 Ask if he is 100% convinced he is a paedophile, i.e. determine if this is of delusional intensity or if there is doubt.

4 Ask how he knows he is a paedophile – is it because he is being 'told' he is a paedophile or did he believe it to be true prior to being told (i.e. is it a primary delusion)?

5 Ask him to provide examples of times when he thinks he has been 'talked about'.

6 Ask if there is presence of thought insertion/thought withdrawal/thought broadcasting.

7 Ask if there is presence of auditory hallucinations.

8 Focus on other Schneiderian first-rank symptoms – 'made' actions/beliefs.

9 Ask whether he thinks the TV or radio communicate to him.

10 Ask about mood symptoms.

11 Ask about risk issues – do these thoughts lead him to do anything to himself or to others?

12 Does he have command hallucinations ordering him to do anything?

13 Assess his insight, i.e. does he believe that he could have a mental illness and what does he believe is the correct treatment for him? Does he believe that he needs hospitalisation or medication?

Discussion

This patient, in distress, has come willingly to your clinic seeking help. These are egodystonic symptoms, therefore this scenario tests empathic history taking and mental state examination. To do well in this scenario, it is advisable to follow the patient's verbal cues and try to summarise your findings with the patient, i.e. try to give feedback to the patient by describing his symptoms back to him in your own words. This will give the examiner the impression that you are empathising with the patient and that you have understood the patient so far. The ability to handle a distressed patient well will score you high marks.

Another aspect to this scenario is evaluating risk and whether his symptoms cause him to behave in a manner that puts children at risk.

Other psychotic phenomenology as well as the patient's own insight also needs to be tested for.

Notes

4a Mrs Baker is meeting you on the ward. Her 19-year-old son, Jake, has been admitted under Section 2 of the Mental Health Act and she wants to know what is likely to happen in the next few days. This is Jake's first presentation. You are unclear about his diagnosis.

INSTRUCTIONS TO CANDIDATES

Explain to Mrs Baker what the short-term management is likely to be, addressing her concerns. Do not take a collateral history.

This is about communicating difficult information to a parent.

Musts

1 Explain to Mrs Baker that he is in hospital as this is currently the safest place for him.

2 Explain the need for PRN medication. Mrs Baker may be hostile to the thought of her son receiving medication forcibly and will need reassurance.

3 Explain that the Mental Health Act has been invoked as a means of keeping him in a safe place while assessment is done and a diagnosis made.

4 Explain what tests will be done, e.g. drug screens.

5 Encourage Mrs Baker to be part of the process and to visit the ward and talk to nursing staff.

Discussion

This is a common scenario for junior doctors on call: a young adult with his first presentation on an acute psychiatric ward. His mother will be faced with many unknowns and needs patience and reassurance from you. This scenario tests how you can manage her anxiety while addressing her concerns in a professional and empathic manner. Try not to 'lecture' her or overload her with information.

Try to give her an overview of the situation, namely that the priority is the safety of her son. She may be aware of some aspects of his behaviour that led to his detention in hospital. The use of medication and rapid tranquilisation needs to be described patiently as she may have preconceived ideas about this.

She may blame herself for the situation, so reassure her by trying to include her as much as possible in her son's management. Encourage her to visit, invite her to the ward round and offer her information sheets.

Notes

4b Jake does not improve and is detained at hospital under Section 3 of the Mental Health Act. The team think he has had a psychotic episode and he is started on olanzepine. After two months he improves and is fit for discharge. His father meets you on the ward to discuss his long-term management.

INSTRUCTIONS TO CANDIDATES

Discuss with Mr Baker his son's long-term management and address his concerns.

This is about knowledge of aftercare.

Musts

1 Explain that Jake needs a long-term strategy.

2 Explain the need for long-term medication to:

    a achieve remission

    b minimise probability of relapse.

3 Explain that Jake's level of engagement and compliance with medication will help his prognosis.

4 Explain the need for the bio-psycho-social approach.

5 Explain the need for a community psychiatric nurse (CPN)/ early intervention service.

6 Explain the need for regular outpatient follow-up.

7 Explain that prognosis can't be predicted.

Discussion

This scenario tests knowledge of aftercare. The patient's father will have plenty of questions about future management. It is important to describe in detail all aspects of management. The bio-psycho-social model is a useful framework to use here. It is important to emphasise that the medication did help him improve and that he needs to stay on medication to prevent relapse. The medication will be reviewed regularly and other professionals can provide support. Do not try to predict prognosis because this is impossible after one episode. Emphasise that constructive engagement with outpatient services and good physical health will improve prognosis.

Notes

5 You are the ward doctor. Alan Marwood is a 30-year-old inpatient on the ward ready for discharge. He has a diagnosis of schizophrenia and has had many admissions in the past. When in hospital he does well and gets better quickly on olanzepine 10 mg/day. However, in the community he relapses easily secondary to non-compliance. Today is his discharge CPA and you are discussing the case with Steve Wilson, his new care coordinator.

INSTRUCTIONS TO CANDIDATES

Discuss the long-term management options with Mr Wilson. Focus on how this cycle of repeated admissions can be minimised.

This is about trying to manage non-compliance in the community.

Musts

1 Discuss barriers to compliance, e.g. substance misuse/poor insight.

2 Discuss the patient's level of engagement with the service.

3 Discuss the patient's support at home – involvement of family – is his home situation stable? Does he need more supported accommodation or to be warden controlled?

4 Discuss community options, e.g. day centres/ancillary organisations, occupational programmes/training – regular CPAs.

5 Discuss the role of depot medication.

6 If the above management strategies are unlikely to be successful discuss the assertive outreach approach.

Discussion

Another common scenario. In this case, you are discussing a patient who does not appear to be making any progress. It is important to try to break this cycle of admission–treatment–recovery–discharge–non-compliance–relapse–admission and to do this you need to explore barriers to compliance in the community. Typically this could be adverse effects of medication, poor insight, a poor relationship with his community mental health team, substance misuse or an unstable home situation. Also the structure of his day needs to be explored. If the patient has no structure then he can disengage from treatment easily and one visit per week from his CPN would not be sufficient to hold him.

Therefore other management strategies, aimed at improving any of the above, need to be discussed. Assertive outreach may be an option. This is a specialist team dealing with patients who engage poorly with their community mental health teams and have spent long periods in hospitals. These patients are regularly visited in their homes so they can be monitored closely in the community to minimise the time they spend as inpatients.

Notes

6 Charlie Robbins is 43 years old and lives in supported accommodation. He has been on a long-acting risperidone depot for several months. He has had several admissions for schizophrenia with predominantly negative symptoms. He has been on olanzepine and aripiprazole in the past without any benefit. He is very susceptible to extrapyramidal side effects. The warden tells you that Mr Robbins has been more withdrawn lately and is refusing to participate in the games activities that he normally enjoys. He is still compliant with his depot and enjoys a good relationship with support staff.

INSTRUCTIONS TO CANDIDATES

You are on a domiciliary visit. Discuss further treatment options with Mr Robbins and his warden. Do not ask about his symptoms.

This is about treatment resistance.

Musts

1 Empathise with Mr Robbins about the fact that his condition has not improved despite being on different medication.

2 Suggest that a different medication could be tried and get his agreement on this.

3 State that clozapine can be tried and outline its potential for benefit, in particular, for negative symptoms.

4 Inform him that the purpose of trying clozapine is to reduce the likelihood of future relapses and lessen the time spent in hospital. Progress can be monitored this way.

5 Advise that an inpatient stay may be the most appropriate place to start clozapine, particularly as it appears he is becoming unwell.

6 Mention regular blood tests and blood sugar monitoring, i.e. weekly for the first three months and tell him that this can be done by a specialist at a clozapine clinic.

7 Mention the side effects of clozapine while stating the advantages.

8 Work hard to get him to agree to an informal admission.

9 Mention the role of CPA aftercare.

Discussion

In this scenario there is a compliant patient who has had an unsuccessful trial of long-acting risperidone constra. Two other atypical antipsychotics (olanzepine and aripiprazole) have been ineffective and typical antipsychotics are contraindicated in view of his susceptibility to neurological side effects.

Therefore clozapine is indicated. This patient lives in supported accommodation and as such will get good support where he lives. Starting clozapine is best done as an inpatient as he is relapsing with evidence of more negative symptoms. On the ward he will be able to receive appropriate blood tests (blood counts) and other investigations, e.g. electrocardiograms (ECGs) and blood pressure monitoring.

Side effects of clozapine include hypersalivation, weight gain and sedation. Progress can be monitored through regular outpatient reviews and CPAs. The benefits can be measured in terms of a reduced need for hospital admission.

Notes

3 Mood disorders

7a Michael Rees, a 35-year-old married salesperson with two children, has been well maintained on citalopram 40 mg/day. He attends outpatients and complains that his sexual performance has been poor lately.

INSTRUCTIONS TO CANDIDATES
Take a history from Mr Rees, trying to establish the cause of his complaint.

This is about not assuming that his sexual dysfunction is connected to citalopram and realising that other causes need to be explored.

Musts

1 Ask him when he first noticed his sexual dysfunction – can he date when it began?

2 Ask him what he means by 'sexual dysfunction' – impotence, anorgasmia, poor libido?

3 Is the sexual dysfunction progressive or did it have a sudden onset?

4 Is he suffering a depressive episode that could be resulting in a loss of libido?

5 Any background medical history? Does he have diabetes, for example?

6 Any substance misuse/alcohol abuse?

7 Does he have any life/work stressors that predate the sexual dysfunction?

8 Does his sexual dysfunction predate citalopram use?

9 Discuss and date when the citalopram doses were increased and whether does increases worsen the sexual dysfunction.

10 Has he had any other problems with citalopram, e.g. gastrointestinal (GI) upset/rash?

Discussion

Although selective serotonin reuptake inhibitors (SSRIs) can cause sexual dysfunction, it is important to understand the temporal sequence, i.e. which of these came first – starting antidepressants or the sexual dysfunction.

It is important to differentiate different types of dysfunction, i.e. has he lost his sex drive or is it impotence/anorgasmia/premature ejaculation? He suffers from depression, which can result in loss of libido. Other potential causes of this dysfunction need to be investigated, e.g. life stressors, relationship difficulties, smoking, alcohol.

This scenario tests also communication skills in managing a patient in distress who may find this subject difficult to talk about.

Notes

7b Mr Rees blames everything on medication and now states vehemently that he won't ever take medication again. He is very interested in psychological treatments and meets you to discuss these options only.

INSTRUCTIONS TO CANDIDATES

Discuss with Mr Rees the common psychological treatments and address his concerns.

This is about communicating how psychological treatments work.

Musts

1 Do not challenge Mr Rees's opinion on medication.

2 Introduce him to talking therapies.

3 Explain that there are a range of different therapies that differ in terms of treatment time and approach.

4 Explain that he will be referred to the psychology department for an initial assessment where these ideas will be discussed further.

5 Introduce common therapies such as cognitive behavioural therapy and psychodynamic psychotherapy.

6 Discuss the differences among them – time limited/problem-based versus gaining insight

7 Discuss with him various lifestyle changes that could improve his condition.

Discussion

In this scenario, this patient has come to clinic wanting to explore psycho-therapies, as there is evidence of their efficacy. He does not want to hear evidence for medication.

His choice between cognitive therapy and psychodynamic psychother-apy depends on a multitude of factors. They include how much time he can spend in therapy and what he wants to achieve from therapy.

Notes

8a

Holly Bailey is a 35-year-old married woman in your out-patient clinic. She has a diagnosis of bipolar affective disorder. She is six weeks pregnant. She was discharged three months ago after a hypomanic episode. In the last five years she has been admitted four times, usually under the Mental Health Act. She is on lithium 400 mg *nocte* and olanzepine 15 mg/day. She is worried about the effects of her medication on the foetus.

She does not want to breastfeed.

INSTRUCTIONS TO CANDIDATES

Discuss management options with Mrs Bailey, addressing her concerns.

Musts

1 Mention to her that if medication is stopped there is a risk that she may relapse, which may impair her ability to care for her unborn child.

2 Mention that the period of maximum risk post-conception with lithium has already passed (two to six weeks). The risk of Ebstein's anomaly is 1:1000. Withdrawal from lithium is therefore not absolutely necessary but if desired must be slow.

3 Mention the need for regular blood lithium level checks (four weekly during pregnancy). Signs of toxicity in the mother may include fluid retention and vomiting.

4 Mention there is little statistically robust evidence, besides a few case reports, that suggests taking olanzepine is dangerous during pregnancy.

5 Mention that due to the increased risk of relapse it is advisable to continue with both lithium and olanzepine, but if lithium is not an option encourage the use of olanzepine at least.

6 Mention that paediatricians should be present at delivery to monitor the foetus' heart if lithium is to be used.

7 Mention that antenatal care coordination is essential and it may be appropriate to involve the obstetrician as well as other involved healthcare professionals, e.g. dietician, GP, midwife. Ultrasound and echocardiography are also essential at six and eighteen weeks should lithium be considered appropriate.

8 Mention the risk of relapse in the post-partum period is eight-fold and that her mental health will be closely monitored by her psychiatric team during this period.

Discussion

This is a classic scenario of a poorly controlled patient who has had four admissions in five years who becomes pregnant. The central issue is to balance the mental health needs of this patient with the risks to the foetus, i.e. if medication is stopped then she may relapse, posing risks to mother and foetus. Therefore discussions will focus around the issues stated above. The major difficulty is that no research can be done on pregnant patients so evidence is based on case reports. British National Formulary (BNF) guidance does not really help, so you have to follow *The Maudsley Prescribing Guidelines.*[*]

---

[*] Taylor D, Paton C, Kapur S.*The Maudsley Prescribing Guidelines*. 10th ed. London: Informa Healthcare; 2009.

Notes

8b   Two weeks ago, Mrs Bailey gave birth to a healthy baby boy but her husband has become increasingly concerned about her mental health. He notices that her self-care has been poor and that she does not seem to be coping. He brings her to your emergency clinic to discuss this.

INSTRUCTIONS TO CANDIDATES
Take a brief history and carry out a mental state examination of Mrs Bailey. Do not discuss management options.

Musts

1 Ask about how she is coping with the baby. In particular, ask about her breastfeeding and sleep.

2 Ask about biological symptoms of a mood disorder, i.e. her energy/mood/sleep and whether there is presence of diurnal mood variation.

3 Ask if she feels tearful/elated.

4 Ask about cognitive symptoms of a mood disorder, i.e. does she have excessively negative or positive opinions about herself, the world or the future?

5 Ask her about suicide/deliberate self-harm ideation, intent or plans.

6 Ask her about presence of mood-congruent psychotic symptoms, e.g. delusions of grandeur/nihilism/hypochondriasis.

7 Ask what her beliefs are about the baby. Are there any abnormal beliefs?

8 Ask about insight and whether she agrees there is something wrong with her mental health. What does she think is the problem and what does she see as the solution?

9 Once you have a general understanding of her mental state, do a risk assessment of the baby's safety.

Discussion

This is a case where a mother has relapsed post-partum and the presentation can be dramatic. Mood symptoms are more likely to contain psychotic features. Try to get a good idea of her mental state before doing a risk assessment because it is more important to build up a rapport first. Initially launching into a risk assessment of the baby's safety may make the mother more hostile and impair your ability to carry out an accurate mental state examination.

The examiners will mark you on how well you carry out a full mental state examination of a distressed patient who may lack insight and hold abnormal views about her baby that may compromise his safety.

Notes

4 Neurotic disorders

9 Angela Reilly is a 45-year-old bank clerk. She has been in trouble at work because she has been persistently late despite living only three miles from her bank. Her boss has told her that she is 'slow'. There have been no complaints about the quality of her work.

INSTRUCTIONS TO CANDIDATES
Interview Ms Reilly to establish the cause of her problems.

Musts

1 Establish what is making her late – is she oversleeping? Is she taking a long time to get ready in the morning? How long does the journey take? How long has she had this problem?

2 Establish what the boss means by her being 'slow'.

3 If she is oversleeping, explore depressive symptomatology.

4 If she is taking a long time to leave the house, explore obsessive symptoms – these would be uncomfortable and intrusive thoughts that she cannot get rid of.

5 If she has these symptoms, does she perform any actions to counter the thoughts? Are there any rituals she has to perform in the morning that may delay her?

6 If she has rituals/actions, ask her if they temporarily relieve anxiety but are in themselves not pleasurable.

7 Does she have any counting or checking rituals?

8 Ask about her insight and what she believes the problem to be. Find out what she sees as the solution.

Discussion

Slowness can be a symptom of different psychopathologies. Depression with psychomotor retardation and obsessive–compulsive disorder (OCD) with rituals need to be investigated. Her age of presentation and her reasonably high level of functioning make a psychotic illness or cognitive impairment unlikely.

Patients with OCD can be embarrassed and ashamed by their symptoms. They often suffer in silence. Try to establish the diagnosis by using the *International Statistical Classification of Diseases and Related Health Problems: 10th Revision* (ICD-10) criteria,* spending an hour per day for two weeks.

---

* World Health Organization (WHO). *International Statistical Classification of Diseases and Related Health Problems.* 10th rev. WHO; 2007. Available at: www.who.int/ classifications/icd/en/ (accessed 20 December 2010).

Notes

10   You are about to see 32-year-old Mark Walsh in your clinic. He has become more withdrawn and socially isolated in the last three months. His GP, who knows him very well, was surprised by this sudden transformation as he had led a fully active life and was socially very confident. Physical illness or substance misuse is not suspected.

INSTRUCTIONS TO CANDIDATES
Interview Mr Walsh to establish the diagnosis.

Musts

1 Ask about whether there has been a particular precipitant event.

2 If a precipitant event has been established, ask him about post-traumatic stress symptomatology – nightmares, flashbacks, hyperarousal states and avoidance symptoms.

3 Ask whether certain sights, smells or sounds can trigger symptoms?

4 Ask what his daily functioning is like, e.g. is he able to work, shop, cook?

5 Inquire about whether he is able to leave the house and how far can he go out.

6 Ask him about his sleep pattern.

7 Inquire whether he is able to drive or use public transport.

8 Inquire about his social supports.

9 Inquire about agoraphobic symptoms, e.g. anxiety symptoms when away from home

10 Inquire about panic symptoms.

11 Ask about depressive symptoms.

12 Assess suicidality.

Discussion

This scenario is difficult because there is a wide differential diagnosis. He could be having a psychotic or depressive episode. However, if a life-threatening, traumatic event can be identified in the history then post-traumatic stress disorder symptoms need to be investigated. These symptoms are often triggered by sights, sounds and smells associated with the trauma. The patient feels like he cannot escape the memory of the traumatic event, particularly when he is having a flashback. The sleep pattern is affected, as he is often afraid to sleep because of nightmares. He becomes hyper vigilant, believing he is in danger most of the time.

Frequently these patients try to cope by avoiding certain situations and becoming more withdrawn. This can exacerbate existing depressive or anxiety symptoms.

Notes

5 Liaison psychiatry

11 Hilda Watson is 62 years old and suffers from chronic back pain. She has no psychiatric history. Her pain management consultant writes to you stating that ten tablets of cocodamol (30:500) per day no longer control her pain and she is requesting stronger opiate-based analgesia. This consultant cannot identify a cause despite extensive surgical investigation and wonders if there is a psychological cause. Mrs Watson agrees to see you. She is able to accept the findings of the investigations. There is no relevant medical history.

INSTRUCTIONS TO CANDIDATES
Take a history from Mrs Watson, trying to establish the cause of her increased need for analgesia. Do not ask about the characteristics of the pain.

Musts

1 Inquire about how long she has been on her cocodamol regime and for how long the regime was effective in controlling the pain.

2 Try to establish at what time of the day her pain starts and what time of the day she takes her prescribed medication. Also try to estimate the relationship between the pain relief and the taking of the medication.

3 Inquire whether she has had any problems with this analgesia. In particular, ask about side effects of opiates, e.g. chronic constipation.

4 Ask about any symptoms of opiate withdrawal, e.g. lacrimation/runny nose/sweats/shakes/diarrhoea.

5 Inquire whether she has self-medicated by giving herself more than the prescribed dose.

6 Inquire about use of other analgesics.

7 Inquire about use of illicit drugs/alcohol.

8 Inquire about depressive symptoms – in particular, cognitive symptoms.

9 Explore her own insight – ask her what she believes is the problem and what she believes is the best solution.

10 Inquire about hypochondriasis – does she believe that there is anything else wrong with her?

Discussion

There are several possibilities here.

The patient could be supplementing her own prescribed cocodamol with other medication/opiates. She would then become more tolerant of her prescribed opiates and would need a higher dose of opiates to achieve the same effect.

It is also necessary to explore the relationship between her pain and the taking of her medication. She may be in constant pain and the prescribed cocodamol may not have any effect. She may be becoming addicted to opiates or chronic constipation could be causing the back pain.

Depression needs to be ruled out. She has risk factors for depression (chronic pain) and exacerbation of pain could be a symptom of depression.

Hypochondriasis could also be a factor. She has had many consultations with her consultant resulting in extensive investigations. She may believe that her back condition is getting worse, which then drives her need for more analgesia. Hypochondriasis can be also a sign of depression.

Notes

12a

Mr Singh, the A&E consultant, is talking to you about Rhianne Foster, a 19-year-old who attended A&E claiming she took an overdose of 100 paracetamol tablets. She has needed Parvolex in the past. Ms Foster is now threatening to leave A&E and states that she wants to die as she sees no future. She is being comforted by nursing staff and is not actively trying to leave. Mr Singh wants you to detain her under Section 2 of the Mental Health Act immediately in case she tries to leave as he suspects a large overdose.

INSTRUCTIONS TO CANDIDATES

Discuss management options with Mr Singh, addressing his concerns.

Musts

1 Try to establish what has happened in the A&E department up to this point. In particular, focus on what measures the A&E staff have taken to keep her in the department, i.e. was hospital security needed? How did A&E staff manage to comfort her? What appeared to be effective?

2 Ask if she is alone or whether she has an adult with her.

3 Try to explain that this is an issue of capacity. If Ms Foster lacks capacity then common law can be used. Capacity can be established by asking the following questions.

   a Does she understand the implications and risks of being treated versus not being treated?

   b Can she trust that the information being given to her is for her own benefit?

   c Can she weigh up all the information to make an informed decision regarding treatment?

4 Explain that an assessment of capacity can be done jointly by the psychiatric doctor and the A&E doctor.

5 Explain that the Mental Health Act can only be invoked in the treatment an underlying mental illness and cannot be used to justify the administration of blood tests for Parvolex treatments.

6 Reassure Mr Singh that you will attend A&E shortly and help him to manage his own anxiety. If Ms Foster becomes acutely restless and tries to leave the department, then using common law to keep her there would be justified as she has taken large overdoses in the past.

7 Mention that your own consultant will be present. This will provide greater reassurance.

Discussion

In this situation it is important to discover what non-coercive actions the A&E staff have done to keep her in the department. Clearly she is ambivalent about wanting to leave the department as the A&E staff have been able to persuade her to stay so far. This ambivalence is actually raising the A&E consultant's anxiety level because all he wants is a clear management plan to free up his nurses. Thus, this scenario tests the ability to communicate with a professional who may have different expectations than you: he is pressing for a more immediate resolution to this ambivalence and you are unable to provide it. Therefore discussion of a cooperative management plan is needed.

Essentially this is about capacity. The psychiatrist and the A&E staff should assess capacity jointly as it is the A&E staff who are providing the medical treatment and the psychiatrist who is assessing her mental state. A patient has capacity if:

1 they can demonstrate they understand the implications of both accepting and refusing treatment

2 they believe that the treatment team are acting in their best interests

3 they are able to give a reasoned argument for their course of action.

The psychiatrist's role in this is to look for signs and symptoms of mental illness that may interfere with her thinking, e.g. she may have delusional beliefs about A&E staff or she may be severely depressed, which may interfere with her judgement.

The Mental Health Act can only be invoked in relation to the treatment of a mental disorder and not an overdose. Common law can be used in this situation.

Notes

12b
Ms Foster settles but remains ambivalent about wanting treatment. She agrees to see you but fears being 'sectioned'.

INSTRUCTIONS TO CANDIDATES
Carry out a risk assessment of Ms Foster.

This is a specific and focused task, so straying outside the remit of this will not be rewarded. Using open questions and empathising with the distressed patient is very important.

Musts

1 Ask about details of overdose.

   a Was there a degree of planning? Did she leave a note, for example?

   b Was there degree of isolation when taking the overdose?

   c Were precautions taken to avoid being discovered?

   d Who called for help?

   e Who made the arrangements for her to go to A&E?

   f Was A&E attendance her choice?

2 Ask her whether she is glad to be alive now.

3 Inquire as to her future plans.

4 Ask if there were any precipitant events, e.g. relationship break-up/ anniversary of an event.

5 Explore for symptoms of mood disorder/psychosis.

6 Inquire about substance misuse.

7 Inquire about her demographic details/living situation.

8 Inquire about protective factors, e.g. whether she has strong supportive relationships.

9 Discuss previous attempts and how these attempts were resolved, i.e. did hospitalisation (medical/psychiatric) follow each previous overdose or did she receive home treatment?

10 Find out about her psychiatric history.

11 When considering the Mental Health Act, you must consider potential risk to self and/or others, thus a discussion centred on the reasons why the Mental Health Act could be invoked should be aimed at alleviating her fears.

Discussion

A very common situation encountered by junior doctors on call, this scenario asks for a risk assessment of the patient, which should include taking a history of what happened before, during and after the overdose. Inquire about precipitant events and planning of the overdose, then find out how the overdose was conducted (in isolation or were friends available) and lastly how the overdose was detected.

The mental state examination should focus on her current suicidal ideation, level of intent and actual plans. Then explore depressive and psychotic symptoms in detail.

Once the current mental state examination has been completed, focus on background risk factors. These would be previous self-harm/suicidal episodes (in particular, those requiring medical treatment), psychiatric history, any drug misuse and homelessness. Also ask about protective factors that discourage her from suicidal thoughts, e.g. supportive relationships.

Notes

6 Forensic psychiatry

13a Wayne Phillips is a 32-year-old prisoner on remand. He has a diagnosis of paranoid schizophrenia and he fatally stabbed a co-resident at the hostel where he lives. You are visiting in the healthcare wing of the prison as a member of the forensic team that covers his catchment area.

INSTRUCTIONS TO CANDIDATES

Take a history around the offence to establish whether his underlying illness had any bearing on this offence. Do not carry out a risk assessment. Do not assess Mr Phillip's fitness to stand trial.

This tests the candidate's knowledge of the relationship between mental disorder and offending.

Musts

1 Find out what Mr Phillips remembers about the offence.

2 Get a history about this offence.

3 Try to establish what Mr Phillip's own justification for the offence is.

4 Establish what the victim did prior to the offence.

5 Establish why this victim was selected.

6 Establish how Mr Phillips was feeling before the offence, i.e. was there a delusional system?

7 Ask about any Schneiderian first-rank symptoms around the time of the offence.

8 If there were symptoms, did they relate to the offence in any way?

9 Ask how he felt after the offence – remorseful? Relieved?

10 Did he have any symptoms after the offence?

11 Determine whether there is any connection between these symptoms and the offence.

Discussion

This scenario may be unfamiliar to many junior doctors. Often patients who have committed these types of violent offences spend long periods of time in custody before being assessed by the forensic teams. In this case, the forensic team are there to assess whether the prisoner's mental illness had a direct relationship to the fatal stabbing. To do this, they need to explore any mental state abnormalities at the time of the stabbing and determine whether these abnormalities contributed directly to the incident. The visiting psychiatrist needs to establish the prisoner's own reasoning and justification for the stabbing and find out why this victim was chosen. It is also possible that the patient may have had acute symptoms that had nothing to do with the offence. Level of remorse and insight also need to be tested.

The mental state examination should focus on Schneiderian first-rank symptoms pertaining to the stabbing.

It is possible that the prisoner's own symptoms and the offence are totally unconnected. In this case, the normal criminal justice route will be taken.

Notes

13b You decide that Mr Phillips was psychotic at the time of his offence and you are discussing the case with your covering consultant, Dr Nash, who is unfamiliar with this case. You suspect that he was non-compliant in taking his olanzepine and this was the reason for his psychosis and that a relapse of his illness directly caused the offence. You also note that Mr Phillips is unwell and is unlikely to be able to stand trial.

INSTRUCTIONS TO CANDIDATES
Discuss with Dr Nash the management options.

This tests knowledge of forensic sections.

Musts

1 Justify your diagnosis of Mr Phillips, explaining why you think he committed the crime, i.e. state that Mr Phillips committed the offence on the victim because of this complex delusional system involving the victim where he believed (the answer the patient gave in the earlier part to this station in 8a, i.e. his delusional system).

2 Explain that Mr Phillips is acutely unwell and needs a hospital transfer under Section 48/49 of the Mental Health Act.

3 Mention that Mr Phillips is currently held under a fairly high level of security, given the nature of his offence, so he may need to be transferred to a medium security facility; he may need to stay on remand until such a vacancy arises.

4 State that in view of his mental disorder and the nature of his offence, he may be given a Section 37/41 'hospital order with Home Office restrictions'.

Discussion

There are two issues here. Firstly, the acute management, in terms of where the prisoner should be managed now, and secondly, the long-term management in terms of how the prisoner needs to be managed in the future.

For the acute management, Section 48/49 of the Mental Health Act allows transfer from prison to a psychiatric hospital for a prisoner who has not been sentenced yet. The prisoner would then be able to receive specialist mental health care that is not available in prison.

Prison healthcare wings manage many people with known mental illnesses. They usually have sessional psychiatrists and full-time nurses. Hospital transfer tends to occur when prisoners are too unwell and cannot be contained in prison.

Given the seriousness of the offence, Mr Phillips would need to be in a medium secure unit in order to contain him. A regular psychiatric hospital would not offer such security. A psychiatric intensive care unit (PICU) would also be insufficient and are usually reserved for a lower level of offence.

For the long-term management, the prisoner needs a high level of mental health input. The visiting forensic team are likely to recommend to the judge that the prisoner serve his sentence in a hospital that can meet his mental health needs. Section 37 allows for this to happen.

This prisoner's offence clearly renders him a risk to others. The use of a restriction order, under Section 41, will keep him in hospital. While in hospital, his level of risk will be monitored regularly and the Ministry of Justice informed of his progress. The Ministry of Justice has the over-riding authority over how and when the prisoner will be released back into the community.

Notes

14 Barry Wilkinson is a 32-year-old informal inpatient with a diagnosis of depression. He is due to attend magistrates' court tomorrow on a charge of handling stolen goods. A custodial sentence is possible. You are the ward doctor.

INSTRUCTIONS TO CANDIDATES
Interview Mr Wilkinson to establish whether he is fit to attend court. Do not ask specifics about the offence.

Musts

1 Introduce yourself to Mr Wilkinson and explain your role.

2 Explain that this interview is not entirely confidential and that some of the findings will be reported to the court.

3 To be considered fit to plead, he must be able to understand and be capable of involvement in the proceedings. Establish whether Mr Wilkinson:

   a understands the nature of the charges

   b understands the implications of a 'guilty' or 'not guilty' plea

   c can instruct the defence

   d can challenge the jurors

   e can follow the court proceedings.

4 Do a current mental state examination of Mr Wilkinson, focusing on depressive symptoms and delusional beliefs, e.g. guilt.

Discussion

A defendant may not be well enough to attend court. This could happen if their mental health deteriorates enough to impair their thinking. If a patient is depressed, they may have delusions of guilt and plead guilty to an offence that they did not commit, feeling that they deserve to be punished.

To evaluate fitness to attend court, the defendant must be able to understand the court proceedings, challenge jurors and instruct the defence. They must also be able to understand the nature of the charges and the implications of a guilty or not guilty plea. A guilty plea refers only to whether he actually committed the offence. Mitigating circumstances will be considered in the sentencing.

Notes

15 You are seeing 28-year-old John O'Neill in outpatients. He has just been released from prison after serving a sentence for street robbery and wants to know if he has a personality disorder because he heard that term in prison. Since the age of 15, he has had over 15 convictions for a variety of offences.

INSTRUCTIONS TO CANDIDATES

Take a history from Mr O'Neill with a view to assessing whether he has a dissocial personality disorder.

This is about building a rapport and asking relevant questions in an empathic way.

Musts

1 Try to establish what Mr O'Neill understands by the term 'personality disorder'.

2 Explain to him that you will need to ask certain questions about his lifestyle to get a more complete picture.

3 Ask about his past forensic history.

4 Ask him if he gets into trouble easily.

5 Ask if he gets easily provoked into fights.

6 Ask how he feels towards his victims.

7 Ask if he feels remorseful about his offences.

8 Ask how he feels about getting into trouble frequently.

9 Ask how he feels about other people in general – whether he has an angry or apathetic attitude towards others.

10 Ask about his employment history, in particular, whether he has been dismissed from jobs.

11 Ask about his relationship history; in particular, look for evidence of casual relationships but no significant long-term ones.

Discussion

Those with a dissocial personality disorder get into conflict with society easily. They are frequently imprisoned, which does not deter them. Such people exist on the margins of society and have often faced family rejection. They have tremendous difficulty holding down jobs or long-term relationships. They are adept at making casual friendships quickly but not at keeping them.

They are often impulsive and take part in risky behaviour. Substance misuse is common.

People with a dissocial personality disorder may possess a hatred or callous disregard for other people and do not express any remorse for their victims.

Often they have had behavioural problems in childhood resulting in exclusion from school.

Notes

7 Psychiatry of older people

16 Christina Stannard is an 81-year-old unmarried woman who has lived in residential care for several years. She has no known contact with psychiatric services. The manager asks you to see Ms Stannard as she has began to refuse food, believing staff are poisoning her. She now only eats food that has been sealed, such as biscuits. Over the last three months she has made many complaints about other staff and residents. Her GP has visited her several times and baseline investigations of her health showed that all aspects of her physical health were within normal parameters.

INSTRUCTIONS TO CANDIDATES

Interview Ms Stannard to establish the diagnosis. Do not perform a cognitive assessment.

Musts

1 Establish onset and course of symptoms.

2 How does she perceive the food being served?

3 Ask if she has a problem with the food or the way it is being served.

4 How does she view staff members – i.e. does she see them as being against her?

5 Ask how she views residents – i.e. does she see them as being against her?

6 Were there precipitating factors? E.g. an event in the home? Problems with any resident/staff member?

7 Inquire about her family. Has there been any news in her family? visits.

8 Ask about any changes in physical health, e.g. hearing loss/neurological deficit.

9 Ask whether there have been depressive symptoms/Schneiderian first-rank symptoms.

Discussion

The aim of this scenario is to elicit as much information about her beliefs about the food and why she is suspicious of it.

There is a wide differential diagnosis. Almost any biological, psychological or social stressor can precipitate a behavioural change in the older person and therefore a broad-based questioning approach is necessary. Ms Stannard is likely to be suspicious of you.

It is possible that she has developed a single delusional system over time that would account for her symptoms. There may not be any other Schneiderian first-rank symptoms.

A depressive episode with psychotic features is also possible. Toxic confusional state is less likely as this would have probably been picked up by the GP.

Notes

17a

Alf Richards is an 85-year-old inpatient on the ward with a diagnosis of depression. The nursing staff call you because he appears to have had a cerebrovascular event with sudden onset right-arm weakness.

INSTRUCTIONS TO CANDIDATES

Examine the cranial nerves and the upper extremities. Avoid corneal reflex, pin prick and jaw jerk.

Engage the patient while examining him.

Musts

1 CNI: Ask about any deficit in sense of smell.

2 CNII: Examine visual fields/visual acuity – use light (if available) to examine direct and consensual pupil reflex.

3 CNIII, IV, VI: Examine his eye movements.

4 CNV: Test facial sensation in three locations or test motor component by asking him to clench teeth while feeling the masseter muscle.

5 CNVII: Raise his eyebrows/puff out his cheeks.

6 CNVIII: Whisper a number between 1 and 100 in each ear.

7 CNXI: Get patient to shrug his shoulders against resistance.

8 CNXII: Examine his tongue movements.

9 Upper limbs: Check tone, power, coordination, reflexes and sensation.

Discussion

It is important to practise neurological examination because it has appeared in MRCPsych exams in the past. The Musts list on the previous page constitutes a shortened version that will cover most areas.

Notes

17b

Mr Richards has 3/5 power on the right side.

INSTRUCTIONS TO CANDIDATES

Examine the cardiovascular system to establish the cause of this event and report your findings to the examiner.

Musts

1 Inspect the patient before examining him.

2 Inspect his fingers and hands for cyanosis/clubbing.

3 Feel his pulse for irregularly irregular pulse.

4 Take his blood pressure – the examiner may tell you to stop.

5 Feel his carotid pulse.

6 Examine his eyes and mouth (for signs of anaemia/dehydration).

7 Feel his apex beat.

8 Auscultate.

Discussion

Atrial fibrillation is a cause of strokes and can be picked up by physical examination. This scenario may present with an ECG that shows no P wave and you could be asked to comment.

Another possible scenario could be demonstrating basic life support on a mannequin, as this is a mandatory yearly requirement of training.

Notes

18 Edith Jenkins, a 76-year-old widow, is an inpatient with a diagnosis of depression. She appears to be deteriorating as her appetite is worsening. Previously she has been on high-dose sertraline, trazodone and venlafaxine on different occasions, but has had little response. No physical cause can be found. The mental health team is considering ECT. Her son wants to talk to you about this.

INSTRUCTIONS TO CANDIDATES

Explain the rationale behind ECT while addressing Mr Jenkins' concerns.

Musts

1 Introduce the topic carefully: 'Good morning, I am Dr X and I would like to discuss your mother's treatment with you.'

2 Explain that Mrs Jenkins' condition has not improved despite medication and that she needs effective treatment to prevent further deterioration.

3 Explain that ECT has been used when medication has not worked.

4 Explain the risk that her depression may get worse unless a new treatment is tried and that worsening depression carries a great risk to her health.

5 Try to elicit her son's knowledge of ECT.

6 Encourage her son to ask questions about the treatment.

7 Explain the procedures of ECT, i.e. 12 treatments, twice a week, under general anaesthetic. The anaesthetic carries a small 1 in 50 000 risk of mortality, which needs to be compared with the risk of a worsening depression.

8 Explain how improvement is assessed and when it is expected.

9 Offer hope by stating that clinical improvement can occur quickly in some cases.

10 Explain the risks and side effects of ECT.

11 Encourage Mr Jenkins to ask further questions.

12 Offer him advice sheets and the contact details of support groups.

Discussion

This patient is deteriorating in hospital and medication is not working. Therefore a new therapeutic approach is needed. Her son will be concerned and may be angry at the hospital, so how you start the meeting is critical.

ECT is a hot topic, but in this case it is strongly indicated because Mrs Jenkins has had treatment failures with three different classes of antidepressants. The mortality risk associated with the use of general anaesthetic is low and it should be considered less of a risk than allowing her depression to deteriorate further.

ECT can cause mild memory deficiencies (anterograde amnesia), but this needs to be placed in the context of what might happen if her depression is allowed to worsen.

The main aim of this scenario is how to overcome people's prejudice about ECT. This can be achieved by outlining the need for ECT in this situation, describing the ECT procedures and stating the risks together with what the clinical expectations could be.

Notes

19a

You are speaking to the husband of Ivy Clifford. She is 86 years old. The GP has referred her to the outpatient department of old-age psychiatry because there have been concerns about her safety. She 'has not been her usual self' over the last three months and she has locked herself out her house on several occasions.

INSTRUCTIONS TO CANDIDATES

Interview Mr Clifford to establish the cause of his wife's problems.

Musts

1 Establish if there have been any precipitants – sometimes external stressors can precipitate worsening functions.

2 Ask about whether she has had any physical health complaints over this time.

3 Establish onset and course of symptoms, i.e. sudden onset or slow onset, gradual deterioration versus stepwise deterioration.

4 Try to assess risk situations, i.e. have keys/money been lost? Gas ovens left on? Has she been wandering?

5 Ask if he feels safe leaving her in the house alone when he goes out.

6 Find out whether she has been disorientated about time, place or person.

7 Ask about any behavioural problems, e.g. crying/shouting.

8 Has he discussed his concerns with his wife and if so how has she responded?

9 Assess how she is coping with the activities of daily living – cooking/shopping/dressing/washing.

10 Establish if there is any evidence of memory loss, e.g. forgetting people's names.

11 Does she talk about any unusual topics that relate to past memories?

12 Has there been evidence of confusion/disorientation/aggression?

13 Ask about whether she has had any depressive symptoms.

Discussion

There are several diagnostic possibilities. These include toxic confusional state, dementia and depression. Toxic confusional state becomes more likely if there is a history of disorientation and clouding of consciousness; dementia becomes more likely if there is evidence of forgetfulness with no clouding of consciousness; and depression is more likely if there is a history of hopelessness, tearfulness and presence of negative cognitions. Clues to her diagnosis will arise from a collateral account of her behaviour. A patient with depression may catastrophise when confronted with a failing memory.

There has been a three-month decline and it is important to distinguish whether the decline has been progressive or stepwise. In stepwise decline, her husband – the collateral historian – can accurately pinpoint when the decline happened. He might say that 'in week one she was able to do X, but in week two she was no longer able to do X'.

The next stage is trying to establish how much her decline has affected their daily lives, focusing on activities of daily living and areas of risk, e.g. loss of keys/leaving a gas oven on – such actions can compromise their safety.

It is also relevant to discover which areas of memory appear to be more affected than most. Long-term memory may function better than short-term memory in a dementing process.

Notes

19b

After a set of routine investigations, psychometric tests and a magnetic resonance imaging (MRI) scan, you diagnose Mrs Clifford with Alzheimer's disease. Her husband has chronic obstructive airways disease and is finding it increasingly difficult to manage her illness. Her MMSE is 19 and you meet with Marjorie, their daughter, to discuss management.

INSTRUCTIONS TO CANDIDATES

Discuss the management of Mrs Clifford with Marjorie, addressing her daughter's concerns.

Musts

1 Explain to Marjorie that her mother has a progressive illness that will affect her memory and her activities in daily living.

2 Explain that there are medical treatments that can slow the progression of the illness but cannot alter the long-term outcome.

3 Explain how these treatments are given and their side effects.

4 Explain how progress is monitored – regular outpatient follow-up.

5 Explain that other professionals may need to be involved, e.g. there may be a role for occupational therapy/social work.

6 Explain that she may need an increase in care packages, e.g. home help.

7 Allow time for her daughter to ask questions.

8 Explain the role that ancillary organisations, e.g. the Alzheimer's Society, can play.

Discussion

The prognosis of Alzheimer's disease, although improved, remains poor. This patient has an MMSE between 10 and 20, which indicates for the use of cholinesterase inhibitors. These medications will delay the disease progression, allowing a greater quality of life. They will not alter the final outcome, which will be a global loss of functioning. All can cause abdominal discomfort due to their pro-cholinergic activity. Arrangements will need to be made to ensure compliance.

Progress on this medication is monitored by three monthly reviews where her MMSE will be tested. If her MMSE falls below 10, then the medication is discontinued.

The bio-psycho-social approach is also needed in the management. Clearly, her husband's failing health may need the involvement of social services who will need to assess her. They would then decide on a package of care based on their findings. They will endeavour to keep her parents maintained in their home as far as possible. However, residential care may have to be considered. This needs to be discussed with her daughter.

The patient should be encouraged to be as mentally and physically active as possible. Consider the use of day centres, crossword puzzles and other activities in the management plan. Discuss information sources such as the Alzheimer's Society.

Notes

8 Child and adolescent psychiatry

20a
Mrs Hemmings attends your Child and Adolescent Mental Health Service (CAHMS) clinic complaining that her 6-year-old son Gareth is aggressive and unpopular with other children. This has been substantiated by his school.

INSTRUCTIONS TO CANDIDATES
Interview Mrs Hemmings to investigate the cause of Gareth's problems.

Musts

1 Ask about their typical home situation.

2 Ask about whether the problem exists in other settings, e.g. playtime/outside classes/social events.

3 Ask about whether he demonstrates inability to focus on one task, e.g. puzzles.

4 Ask about if he is ever hyperactive.

5 Ask about his regularity of sleeping and eating.

6 Ask about the home setting – which adults are in the house?

7 Ask about how Gareth gets on with peers, siblings and adults.

8 Take a developmental history including milestones.

9 Get his medical history.

10 Ask about circumstances around Gareth's birth and Mrs Hemmings' thoughts about the pregnancy.

11 Ask about any medical/psychological difficulties that Mrs Hemmings may have had during pregnancy, postnatally or afterwards.

12 Ask about any periods of separation from Gareth.

Discussion

It is important to determine when and where this 'difficult' behaviour occurs. If the behaviour is restricted to particular situations (i.e. the classroom) then further investigation of Gareth in this environment is warranted, e.g. there may be problems with the teacher or particular pupils.

If, however, this behaviour is pervasive in a multitude of situations, then a diagnosis of hyperkinetic disorder needs to be explored. Hyperkinetic disorder typically results in the affected child being unable to focus or complete a task (e.g. a jigsaw puzzle). This behaviour becomes most obvious at school when they are in a structured organised situation. Other symptoms include restlessness, fidgeting and excessive noisiness in particular situations that require calmness (e.g. during mealtimes, when watching TV). This child may struggle to remain seated in these situations and may be accident-prone. He may eat poorly and have difficulty getting to sleep.

His education and social development will suffer as his behaviour may result in him becoming alienated from his teachers and his peers.

A history of Gareth's home environment is important, focusing on his relationship with all those in his household. A troublesome family life with parenting difficulties can precipitate these symptoms.

Also of relevance is his personal history of his early childhood, as medical illness, family trauma and periods of separation are also risk factors.

Notes

20b

You see Gareth in clinic where he throws all the toys around the room and you arrive at the diagnosis of hyperkinetic disorder. You decide he needs medication and Mrs Hemmings is uneasy about this.

INSTRUCTIONS TO CANDIDATES

Discuss the medication with Mrs Hemmings and address her concerns.

This is about explaining the bio-psycho-social approach as well as medications.

Musts

1 Explain that medication works in conjunction with psychosocial interventions that can be coordinated by parents and teachers.

2 Explain the benefits of medication and what the purpose would be.

3 Explain that medication can be stimulant or non-stimulant.

4 Explain the nature of stimulant (methylphenidate) medication and its side effects.

5 Ask about whether there is a family history of cardiovascular disease.

6 Explain the need for regular monitoring of blood pressure, height and weight to monitor any other potentially harmful interactions.

7 Explain the nature of non-stimulant medication (atomoxetine) and its side effects.

8 Offer Mrs Hemmings some leaflets about the medication and offer her another appointment in a few days so that she has some time to process all the information.

Discussion

It is important to emphasise a multilateral approach to Gareth's management. Interventions are likely to be both pharmacological and non-pharmacological and there will be a treatment plan that involves cooperation among the school, the family, the GP and the CAMHS team. The CAMHS team will explore the family dynamics and consider potential interventions that could be implemented in the home – family therapy may be indicated. Factors at the school may need to be addressed and he may need extra support to achieve educational milestones.

This case is sufficiently serious to consider the use of medication. It is necessary to explain the need for medication in terms of the consequences of not taking medication, i.e. his symptoms may not improve, he will run the risk of falling further behind in his schooling and may suffer further social alienation with the resultant reduction in self-esteem.

There are choices of medication to be offered and the doses are variable according to the level of symptoms. There will be regular reviews and other parameters (height, weight and blood pressure) need to be monitored.

Notes

21 Oliver Brooke is a 16-year-old who has had one admission to hospital – six months ago for a psychotic episode. He recovered on olanzepine. His parents phone the CAMHS team and report that Oliver's behaviour has become more bizarre and that he spends much time in his room drawing disturbing pictures that depict him stabbing his 13-year-old brother with a knife. You are discussing the case with your consultant, Dr Bowers.

INSTRUCTIONS TO CANDIDATES

Discuss the management of this case with your consultant.

This is about assessing the urgency and safety of the situation.

Musts

1 Explain to the consultant the urgency of the situation and the need to see Oliver as soon as possible, taking care to remain safe.

2 Explain the need to involve other team members.

3 Explain the need for telephoning his parents to gauge the level of concern, i.e. does the situation need an urgent full Mental Health Act assessment or a home visit?

4 Explain the need to read his past history and any recent risk assessment.

5 Explain the importance of discussing the domestic situation.

6 Explain that the aim of seeing Oliver is to assess:

   a the level of current risk to self and others

   b his mental state

   c his level of insight.

7 Explain that the outcome will depend on findings but an inpatient admission is possible.

8 Explain the need for exploring the possible reasons for relapse, e.g. non-compliance/substance misuse.

9 Explain the need to take steps to protect the family (especially his brother) and that the family may have to work closely with police and social services to guarantee his brother's safety.

Discussion

This scenario tests your resourcefulness in managing a stressful situation. The consultant will want to see evidence that you can develop a management plan that is comprehensive.

There are three important management aspects: the safety of his younger brother; his deteriorating mental state; and the anxiety of his parents. There may be family dynamics that have exacerbated this situation.

It is important to emphasise cooperative, multidisciplinary working and there may be sufficient concern to warrant a Mental Health Act assessment.

It is also important to discuss risk issues based on past psychiatric history, previous risk history and any background risk factors.

Notes

22a Ray Barnes, a 12-year-old boy, is in your CAMHS clinic because his attendance at school has been poor. His mother is talking to you.

INSTRUCTIONS TO CANDIDATES

Take a history from his mother to investigate Ray's poor attendance.

Musts

1 Find out for how long his school attendance has been reduced and obtain an indication as to how much school time Ray is able to maintain at present.

2 Ask for permission to contact the school to obtain their point of view.

3 Explain to her that school refusal is a symptom rather than a diagnosis, and ask if she knows of any possible reasons why he might be refusing school.

4 Ask if Ray often complains of non-specific physical complaints, e.g. abdominal pain during school days.

5 Screen for disorders such as separation anxiety, phobias (e.g. travelling), bullying, concerns about specific subjects, all global learning deficits, anxiety and agoraphobia, mood disorders, attention deficit hyperactivity disorder (ADHD) and conduct disorder.

6 Differentiate his behaviour from truancy, which is more ego-syntonic, associated with the parents and teachers not knowing where the young person is, may be in a social context with peers, often has a secondary gain and can be associated with some anti-social behaviours.

7 Explain that you would like to meet and assess Ray but will initially need her to be there as chaperone so he will feel more comfortable.

Discussion

There is a need to differentiate school refusal from truancy. Truancy is associated with antisocial behaviour and the whereabouts of the truant person may not be known. School refusal, however, is associated with anxiety, mood disorders, feelings of being inferior to his peers and learning difficulties or phobias. There may be a history of non-specific abdominal complaints.

The context of the refusal is important. Are certain days or lessons being missed or is it pervasive?

Both local and systemic avenues need to be explored. Local causes could include factors in the school, e.g. bullying/a change of teacher.

Systemic causes need to explore the whole family dynamic. There may be a new source of domestic upheaval. There may have been attachment difficulties in childhood that may have been reactivated by this upheaval.

Past psychiatric and medical histories are also important. Time spent in hospital in childhood may have resulted in attachment disorders.

Notes

22b On meeting with Ray he explains to you that he is concerned as he fell behind his work following a period of illness. He feels that he can't catch up and out of place in his peer group who have continued on a fuller schedule. He no longer goes to school as he can't face falling further behind.

INSTRUCTIONS TO CANDIDATES

Explain to Ray's mother your management plan to reintroduce him to school.

Musts

1 Suggest to Ray's mother that he should be reintroduced into school on an agreed temporary part-time schedule to desensitise him to his anxiety of returning, and that this will gradually build up his confidence.

2 State that you will liaise closely with the teachers so they are agreed on his new part-time schedule and can praise and encourage him.

3 If this is initially unsuccessful, suggest that consideration be given to having Ray taught in a small classroom environment, either within the school or in the local hospital's paediatric ward (to encourage socialising within a peer group).

4 Explain that the most extreme option would be some home tuition, which would allow Ray to increase his confidence academically, but would be less helpful in reintegrating him into his peer group).

5 Encourage social activities out of school to increase his confidence.

6 Explore the possibility of a reward programme at home and school, to encourage Ray to go back to full-time schooling.

Discussion

Reintegration back into school needs a multilateral approach. The school, CAMHS and possibly the educational psychologist need to plan a gradual reintroduction that addresses particular concerns.

If attempts to reintegrate him into school are unsuccessful, then home tuition may be the best option.

Efforts need to focus on boosting social confidence with his peers. Encourage participation in sports. Family therapy may also be of benefit. The emphasis should be on building up self-esteem through praise and positive reinforcement.

Notes

23 A GP has referred a 9-year-old girl to you. Her parents are concerned that she is not fitting in with her peers at school even following a change of school when she was 7 to see if this may have helped. Her school notes that she is particularly good at working in some subjects but becomes distressed and performs poorly in others. She cannot cope with group work and often gets detentions for 'silly behaviours'.

INSTRUCTIONS TO CANDIDATES

Take a history from the family to ascertain if she is on the autistic spectrum.

Musts

1 Inquire about how she interacts and plays with others/peers/siblings. Does she play alongside or along with others?

2 Ask about the precipitants of the 'silly behaviours'.

3 Ask about the presence of stereotypes, e.g. same facial expressions.

4 Ask whether she has a narrow range of interests and activities.

5 Ask about her performance in sports.

6 Ask if minor changes in the environment trouble her, e.g. changing the arrangement of furniture.

7 Ask how long the problem has been apparent and whether the behaviour is restricted to a particular situation or whether it is pervasive in all situations.

8 Get a developmental history from birth and ask about developmental delays, e.g. speech.

9 Ask about medical history.

10 Ask if there is a family history of autism.

11 Ask for permission to contact the school to get their feedback.

12 Suggest that the child attends clinic for a multidisciplinary assessment.

Discussion

Children with a mild autistic disease may flourish in certain subjects and struggle in sports and group activities. They may have difficulty reading social situations and enjoy a narrow spectrum of activities. They enjoy sameness and are troubled by interruptions to routine. Often there is a history of delayed developmental milestones. The child may be of a short stature.

Sometimes parents may be able to recall aspects of the child's earlier life and may remember having difficulties in the bonding/attachment process.

Parents may feel guilty and blame themselves, so efforts need to be made to reassure them that this is a recognisable condition that can be managed but not cured.

Notes

9 Risk management scenarios

24a David Peacock agrees to see you in outpatients because he fears what he might do to his wife. He punched his wife in the face recently, claiming that he had heard voices stating she is regularly unfaithful. They have been married for over 15 years and this problem has been present for the last month. He is 45 years old.

INSTRUCTIONS TO CANDIDATES
Interview Mr Peacock to establish the diagnosis.

Musts

1 Explore with Mr Peacock the basis of his belief that his wife has been regularly unfaithful and, in particular, the way his belief has developed over time. This may show a development of a delusional system over time.

2 Ask about whether he has made attempts to prove his wife's unfaithfulness, e.g. cross-examining her, examining her underwear and sexual organs, listening to telephone conversations, following her and assaulting her to extract a confession.

3 Inquire about symptoms characteristic of psychiatric disorders that can result in secondary morbid (not necessarily delusional) jealousy, e.g. schizophrenia, affective disorder, obsessional and other neurotic disorders, alcoholism or other substance abuse.

4 Inquire about their marital and sexual relationship, e.g. is there any history of impotence?

5 Inquire about previous relationships, e.g. is there evidence in these of excessive jealousy/violence?

6 Inquire about previous personality, e.g. is there evidence of low self-esteem/feelings of insecurity/a jealous or paranoid personality?

Discussion

Morbid jealously can be secondary to many psychiatric disorders and may resolve if the underlying psychopathology is treated.

It is important to explore the phenomenology here; whether this belief of infidelity is a delusion, a preoccupation or an obsession. This belief may be heightened by alcohol intoxication. The next stage is to elicit the existence of other associated beliefs and to see how these beliefs are connected. There may be 'knight's move thinking' among beliefs, suggestive of a psychotic process. There may also be evidence of delusional perceptions, e.g. 'I see that my wife is wearing brown, which means she has cheated on me already'.

Once his belief system is better understood, then the risk assessment takes place, i.e. how far does his belief system dictate his actions in trying to 'prove his wife's infidelity'? These actions of course place her at risk.

A background history, exploring risk factors, is also important. Especially his previous relationship history, forensic history and whether there is any evidence of a paranoid, borderline, dissocial or dependent personality disorder.

Notes

24b

Mrs Peacock rings the duty worker at the CMHT. She has moved out of the house after her husband struck her while she was on the telephone speaking to the builder. She states that her husband believed she was speaking to her 'lover' and would accept no other explanation. She expresses fear for her own safety.

INSTRUCTIONS TO CANDIDATES

You are the doctor for this CMHT. Discuss your management of this situation with Mike Evans, the lead social worker for the CMHT, and Shirley Robinson, the consultant psychiatrist.

The priority is to protect Mrs Peacock from serious harm from her husband.

Musts

1 Suggest to Mr Evans, the lead social worker, that a social worker or another appropriate professional be allocated to support the wife, independent of those attempting to treat her husband, one of the reasons for this being to ensure she is in a safe place where she cannot be at serious risk from Mr Peacock, e.g. residing with friends or relatives/in a refuge.

2 Ask that the professional supporting the wife interview her to clarify the history of developing jealousy and violence. The professional should indicate to Mrs Peacock the possibility that mental disorder is the cause of her husband's behaviour and advise on the action to be taken if Mr Peacock confronts her, e.g. call the police.

3 Present the case to Dr Robinson, the consultant psychiatrist, and suggest that a formal Mental Health Act assessment of Mr Peacock be considered with a view to confirming whether he has a mental disorder that requires his detention in hospital for the protection of others or whether he can be safely managed in the community, e.g. if he has the insight to comply with the anti-psychotic medication treatment for morbid delusional jealousy or psychiatric treatment for any psychiatric disorder present.

4 Discuss whether a Multi-Agency Risk Assessment Conference (MARAC) should be convened to manage the risk to Mrs Peacock.

5 Explain that if Mr Peacock's underlying mental disorder is treated then Mrs Peacock will not be so threatened by Mr Peacock's delusional belief system.

Discussion

This is an uncommon scenario that needs multidisciplinary teamwork.

The two major areas of focus are keeping the wife safe and treating his illness. Keeping her safe will involve establishing a place of safety for her and close liaison with police, social services and multi-agency protection panels (MAPPA). It may be better to involve two different social workers: one to work with Mrs Peacock and one to work with Mr Peacock.

If the husband has insight and will comply with an agreed treatment plan, then home treatment teams may be the optimal management plan. These teams, often called 'crisis teams', work closely with patients in their own homes so that admission can be avoided. It is better that the patient works cooperatively with a crisis team than coercively under the Mental Health Act because the more insight the patient has, the better the prognosis.

Detention under the Mental Health Act would be necessary if insight is poor and risk to others remains sufficiently high.

Notes

25 You are speaking to the consultant obstetrician Mr Hussain. He tells you that Marie Walker, a 30-year-old patient with paranoid schizophrenia that you know, saw him earlier today requesting a termination of pregnancy. She is ten weeks pregnant. You know that Ms Walker is in a stable relationship and has tried very hard to get pregnant for the last two years. Mr Hussain tells you that Ms Walker claims that she has 'the son of the devil inside her' and needs to stop the pregnancy to save the world.

INSTRUCTIONS TO CANDIDATES
Discuss management options with Mr Hussain.

Note: The Court of Appeal ruled in 1988 that a foetus is not a person with legal rights.

Musts

1 Suggest to Mr Hussain that the patient may lack the capacity to consent to the termination, as her ability to believe the information she has been given may be interfered with by her delusional thinking.

2 Explain that if it is accepted the patient currently lacks capacity (i.e. is incompetent) to make a decision about a termination, medical staff should act in her best interests and proceed in the way that she is likely to have decided if competent, i.e. she has been trying very hard to become pregnant for the last two years, indicating that she wishes to have a child.

3 Suggest to Mr Hussain that, as you know the patient, you will arrange for an urgent reassessment of her mental state to determine whether she requires additional psychiatric treatment and, if so, whether she will voluntarily accept this or will require a formal Mental Health Act assessment with a view to detention in hospital on grounds of her health and possibly safety.

4 Explain that while antipsychotic medication is best avoided during pregnancy, the possible risks of such medication, including increased extrapyramidal side effects (EPS) in a baby born to a mother given antipsychotic medication in the third trimester, are likely to be outweighed by the risks of not treating the patient. Olanzapine may be a reasonable choice.

5 Advise that additional information may be usefully obtained from the patient's partner, but this ideally requires the patient's consent for him to be approached.

6 Tell Mr Hussain that if the patient fails to adequately respond to psychiatric treatment and there remains a serious risk to Ms Walker due to her delusional beliefs, termination to prevent further deterioration in her mental state, which has associated increased risk to herself, may have to be reconsidered.

Discussion

This is about whether a 30-year-old female patient who suffers from paranoid schizophrenia has the capacity to consent to the termination of a pregnancy and whether she requires additional psychiatric treatment of her mental illness, if necessary compulsorily under the Mental Health Act 1983.

Capacity is best assessed jointly by the psychiatric team and the obstetric team. Capacity is specific to a particular procedure and cannot be generalised, i.e. a patient can have capacity for one procedure but not another. A patient has capacity to consent to a procedure if she can adequately explain the advantages and disadvantages of having the procedure versus not having the procedure. In this case, her explanation of the advantages of the procedure is delusional.

She needs an urgent assessment of her mental health. She may attempt to harm herself to abort the pregnancy. Once again the choice of management depends on her symptoms, her insight and her risk. The spectrum of options, from most mild to most severe, includes outpatient management with CPN involvement, home treatment teams or detention under the Mental Health Act. Olanzepine may be a safer choice of antipsychotic.

Notes

Index